A NO NONSENSE QUICKGUIDE TO

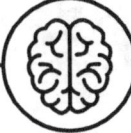

LIVING WITH DIABETES

BY
R. MURDOCH RESEARCH JOURNALISM

A NO NONSENSE QUICKGUIDE TO
LIVING WITH DIABETES

Published by: **Murdoch I/S**, Denmark

No part of this publication may be reproduced, distributed, or transmitted in any form or by any means, including photocopying, recording, or other electronic or mechanical methods, without the prior written permission of the publisher, except in the case of brief quotations embodied in critical reviews and certain other non-commercial uses permitted by copyright law. For permission requests, please contact the publisher at the address below.

Contact: **Murdoch I/S** - rasmus.murdoch@gmail.com

LIMIT OF LIABILITY/DISCLAIMER:

The information contained in this ebook is for informational and educational purposes only. It is not intended as a substitute for professional medical advice, diagnosis, or treatment. Always seek the advice of your physician or other qualified healthcare provider with any questions you may have regarding a medical condition. Never disregard professional medical advice or delay in seeking it because of something you have read in this ebook.

The author and publisher make no representations or warranties with respect to the accuracy, applicability, fitness, or completeness of the contents of this ebook. They disclaim any responsibility for errors or omissions and assume no liability for any loss or damage resulting from the use of the information contained herein. Reliance on any information provided in this ebook is solely at your own risk.

The recommendations in this ebook are intended for general educational purposes and may not be suitable for everyone. Always consult with a healthcare professional before making any changes to your diet, exercise routine, or medical regimen.

A NO NONSENSE QUICKGUIDE TO
LIVING WITH DIABETES

TABLE OF CONTENTS

- **Introduction**: Welcome to Your Diabetes Journey
- **Chapter 1**: Understanding Diabetes
- **Chapter 2**: Coming to Terms with Your Diagnosis
- **Chapter 3**: Building Your Diabetes Care Team
- **Chapter 4**: Monitoring and Managing Your Blood Sugar
- **Chapter 5**: Eating Well with Diabetes
- **Chapter 6**: Exercise for a Healthy Lifestyle
- **Chapter 7**: Medication and Insulin Management
- **Chapter 8**: Managing Complications and Staying Healthy
- **Chapter 9**: Emotional and Mental Well-being
- **Chapter 10**: Living a Full Life with Diabetes
- **Chapter 11**: Building Long-term Healthy Habits
- **Chapter 12**: Moving Forward with Confidence
- **Final Thoughts**: Your Life, Your Journey
- **References**

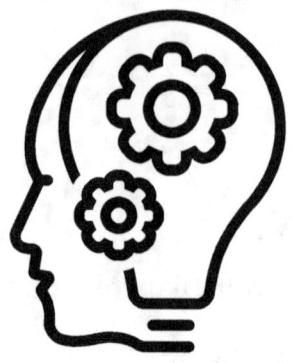

CHAPTER 1:
UNDERSTANDING DIABETES

WHAT EXACTLY *IS* DIABETES?

So, you've been diagnosed with diabetes. First of all—take a deep breath. This is not the end of the world. You're still you, just with a few extra things to keep an eye on. You're about to embark on a journey, and while it may have some bumps (okay, maybe more like potholes), this book is here to help you steer around them.

Let's roll up our sleeves and tackle this head-on. So, what's diabetes all about? Why has your pancreas chosen to kick back and go on a seemingly permanent coffee break?

In simple terms (because we don't need a medical degree to understand our bodies, right?), diabetes is when your body can't properly handle sugar. Normally, you eat something, your body breaks it down into glucose (aka sugar), and your pancreas releases this handy little hormone called insulin to help that glucose get into your cells, giving you energy. But with diabetes, your body either isn't making enough insulin or isn't using it well enough. So, all that sugar just hangs out in your bloodstream, causing trouble—kind of like leaving a bunch of kids unsupervised in a candy store.

Let's break down the types of diabetes:

Type 1 Diabetes: The All-or-Nothing Type

Type 1 diabetes is like that friend who never does things halfway. It usually shows up in childhood or early adulthood, and it's an autoimmune disease. This means your immune system—usually the good guy that fights off germs—gets confused and attacks the cells in your pancreas that make insulin. So, your body just stops making insulin altogether. If you've got Type 1, insulin injections are your new best friend.

But don't worry—people with Type 1 diabetes live long, healthy, active lives. Sure, you have to manage insulin like a pro, but you can still do everything you did before, from running marathons to eating pizza (with a bit of planning, of course).

Type 2 Diabetes: The Procrastinator

Type 2 diabetes is a bit more common—it's the one that tends to sneak up on you over time. Your body is still making insulin, but your cells start ignoring it, like a toddler who won't listen to instructions. This is called insulin resistance. Eventually, your pancreas gets worn out from trying so hard to keep up, and it slows down production.

Type 2 is often linked to lifestyle factors like diet, weight, and exercise, but your genetics can also play a big part. The good news is that Type 2 can often be managed (and sometimes even reversed) with changes to your lifestyle. It's like your body saying, "Hey, let's make some better choices here."

Gestational Diabetes: The Surprise Visitor

If you've ever had a surprise houseguest, you know the feeling of gestational diabetes. It shows up during pregnancy and makes things a bit more complicated. It usually goes away after the baby is born, but having it can increase your chances of developing Type 2 diabetes later. So, it's like a little heads-up from your body to stay mindful of your health.

HOW DID I GET HERE?

Now you might be thinking, "Why me? Did I eat too much ice cream? Did I ignore my mom when she told me to eat my veggies?" Relax. There's no one thing that causes diabetes, and it's definitely not your fault. For Type 1, it's mostly genetic, and for Type 2, it's a mix of genetics and lifestyle factors. Sure, having a healthy diet and staying active can help, but even people who do everything "right" can still get diabetes. So, don't beat yourself up.

WHY IS HIGH BLOOD SUGAR A BIG DEAL?

Okay, so your blood sugar is high. What does that mean? Well, when sugar just sits in your bloodstream instead of going into your cells to be used as energy, it starts causing damage—kind of like leaving milk out on the counter. It messes with your blood vessels, nerves, and organs, which is why controlling your blood sugar is so important.

Uncontrolled diabetes can lead to complications like heart disease, kidney problems, and vision loss, but here's the thing: with good management, you can avoid most of these. The goal is to keep your blood sugar in check so you can live your life without worrying about these issues sneaking up on you.

TAKEAWAY: YOU'VE GOT THIS!

If all this information feels like a lot to take in, that's okay. Managing diabetes is a marathon, not a sprint. You don't have to learn everything in one day. As we go through this book, I'll walk you through everything you need to know about living with diabetes in a way that's easy, manageable, and maybe even a little fun (yes, I said fun). So, grab a snack (we'll talk about what kinds of snacks later) and get ready to take control of your health.

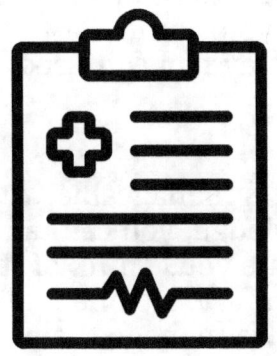

CHAPTER 2:
COMING TO TERMS WITH YOUR DIAGNOSIS

THE EMOTIONAL ROLLERCOASTER

So, you've got diabetes. If you're anything like most people, you've probably gone through the five stages of grief. First, there's denial: "There's no way I have diabetes. The doctor must have switched my blood test with someone else's." Then there's anger: "What did I do to deserve this?!" Bargaining may have sounded like: "Okay, I'll give up ice cream forever if this just goes away!" Depression: "Why even bother eating healthy if I have this condition?" And finally, acceptance: "Okay, I've got diabetes. Now what?"

Here's the thing: no matter what stage you're in right now, it's okay. Diabetes can feel like a tidal wave at first. Suddenly, you're diving into a world of new routines, with doctor visits popping up like they're the new Friday night hangout, and blood sugar checks becoming as frequent as coffee breaks. It's a lot to handle. But here's the good news: you're not alone, and feeling all of these emotions is completely normal. In fact, it's probably healthier to feel them and work through them than to ignore them. The key is to get to a point where you accept the diagnosis and are ready to take control of your health—on your own terms.

GETTING OVER THE SHOCK

Let's be real: when you first hear the words, "You have diabetes," it can feel like someone pulled the rug out from under you. Whether you had a suspicion because diabetes runs in your family or the diagnosis came out of nowhere, it's still a shock. You may feel confused, scared, or even a little angry. All of that is valid.

But here's the thing: diabetes is manageable. Yes, it's a serious condition, but with the right tools and knowledge, you can take control of your health. You don't have to let diabetes define you. Think of it this way: it's just a part of your life now, like taxes or laundry. No one really enjoys dealing with them, but they're a part of life, and we manage them.

YOU'RE NOT ALONE

One of the first things to remember is that you're not alone in this. Millions of people are living with diabetes, and they're thriving. Whether you know it or not, people in your community, at work, or even in your own family are also living with diabetes. Some of them may be doing such a good job managing it that you'd never even know. And with all the resources available today—books (like this one!), support groups, online communities, podcasts—there's always help available.

Finding others who share your experience can be incredibly helpful. Maybe you'll meet someone at your doctor's office, or maybe you'll join an online diabetes community. Talking to people who get it can make all the difference. It's comforting to know you're not the only one dealing with finger pricks and carb counting.

OWNING YOUR DIAGNOSIS

One of the most empowering things you can do is take ownership of your diagnosis. This doesn't mean you have to throw yourself into researching every scientific detail about diabetes, but it does mean taking responsibility for your health. You've got this. You can learn how to manage your blood sugar, adjust your diet, and still live an amazing life.

Some people feel ashamed or embarrassed about having diabetes. They think it's their fault or something they should have prevented. Let me be clear: diabetes isn't about blame. Whether you've been diagnosed with Type 1, Type 2, or gestational diabetes, it's not something you brought on yourself. Sure, there are lifestyle factors involved with Type 2 diabetes, but genetics play a big role too. Plus, blaming yourself won't help—it just wastes time and energy that could be better spent learning how to live your best life with diabetes.

Owning your diagnosis means making peace with it. It's like saying, "Okay, diabetes. You're here. I see you. But you don't get to run the show." The more you accept that you have diabetes and that you can control it, the more empowered you'll feel.

BREAKING THE NEWS TO OTHERS

Now that you've come to terms with your diagnosis (or at least you're getting there), you might be wondering, "Do I have to tell people?" Well, that's up to you.

Some people feel more comfortable keeping their diagnosis private, while others find it helpful to share it with friends, family, or even coworkers. There's no right or wrong here—it's about what makes you feel comfortable.

That said, telling the people closest to you can be helpful, especially in terms of emotional support. Your loved ones might not fully understand what diabetes entails, but they can support you as you learn to manage it. Plus, they can be your cheerleaders when you're having a tough day or when you make great progress.

As for coworkers or acquaintances, that's a personal decision. You might feel it's easier to explain why you're suddenly more conscious of your food choices or why you're checking your blood sugar at your desk. Or, you might not want to bring it up at all—and that's totally fine too.

OVERCOMING FEAR OF THE UNKNOWN

Let's talk about the elephant in the room: fear. It's normal to be afraid when you're diagnosed with diabetes. Fear of complications. Fear of needles. Fear of the unknown. But here's the thing—fear usually comes from not understanding something fully.

The more you learn about diabetes, the less scary it becomes. Knowledge is power. The more you understand how blood sugar works, what foods are good for you, and how exercise can help, the more confident you'll feel. And that confidence will replace a lot of that fear.

And remember, you don't have to learn everything at once. Take it one step at a time. Start with the basics (which, lucky for you, is exactly what this book is all about). As you grow more familiar with managing diabetes, your fear will fade, and you'll feel more in control.

FINDING YOUR MOTIVATION

Living with diabetes requires making changes—no way around that. But it's important to remember why you're making those changes. What's your motivation?

Maybe it's staying healthy for your kids or grandkids. Maybe it's being able to keep doing the things you love, like traveling, playing sports, or enjoying a good meal with friends. Whatever your reason, keep that in mind. It's not about "being good" or following a bunch of rules just because. It's about taking care of yourself so you can live the life you want, diabetes and all.

TAKEAWAY: EMBRACE THE JOURNEY

Coming to terms with your diabetes diagnosis is a process. You won't wake up tomorrow feeling completely at peace with it, and that's okay. But little by little, you'll learn to accept it, manage it, and ultimately live well with it. This is your journey—own it, embrace it, and know that you're stronger than you think.

In the next chapter, we'll talk about **building your diabetes care team**—because no one said you have to do this alone!

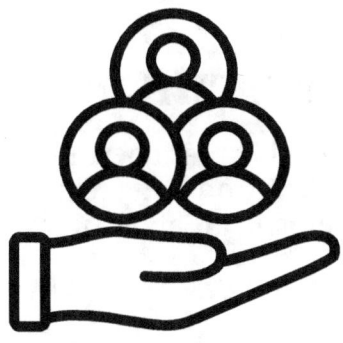

CHAPTER 3:
BUILDING YOUR DIABETES CARE TEAM

YOU DON'T HAVE TO DO IT ALONE

Sure, managing diabetes is something you'll do day-to-day, but here's the good news: you don't have to do it all by yourself. Consider yourself the captain of Team You, with a bunch of experts ready to back you up. Each one has their own superpower, helping you stay on top of diabetes like a champ. It's like assembling a squad of specialists who know how to tackle every twist and turn.

So, who's on your team? Let's break it down.

YOUR PRIMARY CARE DOCTOR: THE QUARTERBACK

Your primary care doctor (PCP) is the first person in your diabetes team. They're like the quarterback in football—they call the plays, direct you where you need to go, and coordinate your care. They probably diagnosed your diabetes in the first place, and they'll help monitor it over time, checking your blood sugar levels, blood pressure, cholesterol, and all that fun stuff.

Your PCP will also refer you to other specialists as needed, so make sure you feel comfortable asking them any and all questions. They're your go-to person for the big picture of your health. You don't have to see them every time your blood sugar spikes a bit, but they'll keep track of your overall progress.

ENDOCRINOLOGIST: THE DIABETES SPECIALIST

Not everyone with diabetes needs an endocrinologist, but if your PCP recommends one, they'll be a key player on your team. Endocrinologists specialize in hormones, and since diabetes is all about insulin (a hormone), these docs know their stuff.

An endocrinologist can help with things like fine-tuning your medications, recommending insulin options, or managing more complex cases of diabetes. If you're struggling with blood sugar control or your medication needs adjusting, they'll step in with expert advice. Endocrinologists are the diabetes pros who can help you get into the details when needed.

DIETITIAN: YOUR FOOD GURU

If you're wondering, "What can I eat now?" the dietitian is your new best friend. A registered dietitian who specializes in diabetes will help you figure out a meal plan that works for your lifestyle and health goals. They'll teach you about carbs, portion control, and how different foods affect your blood sugar. But don't worry—they won't make you give up your favorite foods forever (phew!).

The key with a dietitian is personalization. There's no one-size-fits-all diabetes diet. Your dietitian will help you figure out what works best for you, whether it's finding healthy alternatives, learning how to count carbs, or even just creating a balanced grocery list. They make food fun again (and healthy too!).

DIABETES EDUCATOR: THE TEACHER YOU ALWAYS NEEDED

Diabetes educators (also called Certified Diabetes Care and Education Specialists, or CDCES) are exactly what they sound like—people who educate you on all things diabetes. They're trained to teach you the ins and outs of managing the condition. If you're new to diabetes or still feel confused about things like how to use a glucose meter or how to inject insulin, this is the person who'll walk you through it, step by step.

They'll also help with things like setting realistic goals, problem-solving when your blood sugar goes crazy, and even understanding how stress or illness affects diabetes. In short, they're there to empower you with the knowledge you need to manage diabetes confidently.

PHARMACIST: YOUR MEDICATION EXPERT

Don't forget about your pharmacist! They're a great resource when it comes to medications—whether it's oral meds, insulin, or anything else. Your pharmacist can explain how your meds work, what side effects to watch out for, and how to take them properly.

And since diabetes often comes with other conditions (like high blood pressure or cholesterol), your pharmacist can help you manage multiple prescriptions, making sure everything works together. They might also know about discounts or generic versions of medications, which is always a plus.

EYE DOCTOR: KEEPING YOUR VISION CLEAR

People with diabetes need to keep an eye (pun intended) on their vision. High blood sugar can damage the blood vessels in your eyes, leading to problems like diabetic retinopathy. This is why regular eye checkups with an ophthalmologist or optometrist are important. They'll keep an eye (there's that pun again) on your eye health and catch any problems early.

Don't skip those annual eye exams—even if your vision seems fine. It's much better to catch issues before they cause major problems.

PODIATRIST: FOOT HEALTH IS NO JOKE

Feet? Yes, feet. It turns out, diabetes can affect your feet in ways you might not expect. High blood sugar can damage the nerves in your feet (this is called neuropathy), making it hard to feel pain or injuries. Plus, it can slow down healing, which means a small cut can turn into a bigger issue if it's not taken care of.

That's where the podiatrist comes in. They specialize in foot health and will make sure your feet are in good shape. Whether it's helping with toenail issues, checking for sores, or making sure your shoes fit well, podiatrists are an essential part of your diabetes care team.

MENTAL HEALTH PROFESSIONAL: TAKING CARE OF YOUR MIND

Living with diabetes can be stressful—no doubt about it. Between managing blood sugar, keeping up with doctor's appointments, and making lifestyle changes, it's easy to feel overwhelmed. That's why having a mental health professional on your team is so valuable.

Whether it's a therapist, counselor, or social worker, talking to someone about the emotional side of diabetes can be a huge help. They can help you manage stress, deal with anxiety or depression, and give you coping strategies when diabetes starts to feel like too much.

There's no shame in seeking help for your mental health. In fact, it's one of the smartest things you can do. Remember, your mental health is just as important as your physical health.

SUPPORT NETWORK: YOUR FRIENDS AND FAMILY

Last but definitely not least, let's talk about your personal support network—your friends, family, partner, coworkers, or anyone else who's there for you. These are the people who'll help you navigate life with diabetes, even if they don't fully understand what it's like.

Whether it's reminding you to check your blood sugar, cooking a healthy meal together, or just being there to listen when you're frustrated, your support network plays a huge role in your success. Don't be afraid to lean on them—they want to help, and you'll need them.

TAKEAWAY: ASSEMBLE YOUR DREAM TEAM

Managing diabetes isn't a solo sport. It's more like a team effort, and you're the captain. You've got doctors, specialists, and loved ones all there to help you stay healthy and thrive. Don't be afraid to reach out to them when you need support—because with the right team, you can handle anything diabetes throws your way.

Next up, we'll dive into the nitty-gritty of **monitoring and managing your blood sugar**—because keeping those levels steady is the key to feeling your best.

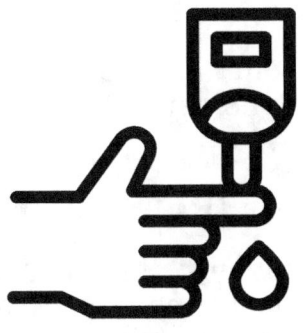

CHAPTER 4:
MONITORING AND MANAGING YOUR BLOOD SUGAR

BLOOD SUGAR: THE BASICS

Ah, blood sugar—the thing you never knew you'd have to think about so much. But here you are, ready to become the boss of your blood sugar. It's time to understand why it matters, how to keep it in check, and what tools can make your life a little easier.

So, what is blood sugar? In simple terms, it's the amount of sugar floating around in your bloodstream. Your body uses this sugar, or glucose, as fuel. When you have diabetes, your body either can't make enough insulin (Type 1) or can't use insulin properly (Type 2). Insulin is like a key that helps glucose get into your cells. Without enough insulin, glucose can't get where it needs to go, so it just hangs out in your blood, causing trouble.

To manage diabetes well, you want to keep your blood sugar within a certain range. The name of the game is balance. Let your blood sugar spike too high, and you're looking at sluggish days and potential long-term trouble. Let it dip too low, and you're in the dizzy zone, possibly heading for an unwanted nap on the floor.

TOOLS FOR MONITORING BLOOD SUGAR

Let's talk tools. Monitoring your blood sugar is a bit like checking the weather: it helps you decide what to do next. Here are your two main options:

1. Blood Glucose Meters (BGMs): The Classic

The tried-and-true method for checking blood sugar is the blood glucose meter. It's simple: you prick your finger, place a drop of blood on a test strip, and voila—your blood sugar reading pops up on the screen. BGMs are reliable, easy to carry, and get the job done. However, they do require finger pricks, which might not be anyone's favorite thing.

2. Continuous Glucose Monitors (CGMs): The High-Tech Solution

If finger-pricking sounds like a drag, consider a Continuous Glucose Monitor (CGM). These nifty devices stick to your skin and check your blood sugar every few minutes, sending the data to your phone or a receiver. It's like having a tiny, invisible assistant constantly monitoring your blood sugar. CGMs can alert you if your levels get too high or too low, which is great for peace of mind.

- **Pros of CGMs:** No finger pricks, real-time data, and the ability to see trends over time.

- **Cons of CGMs:** They can be pricey, and the sensor must be changed regularly.

Both BGMs and CGMs have their pros and cons, so it's all about what works best for you. Either way, the important thing is to keep tabs on your blood sugar.

UNDERSTANDING TARGET RANGES

Okay, so you're checking your blood sugar, but what numbers are you aiming for? Your doctor will give you specific targets, but here's a general idea:

- **Before meals:** 80-130 mg/dL

- **1-2 hours after meals:** Less than 180 mg/dL

- **A1C (your average blood sugar over three months):** Less than 7%

Everyone's targets are a bit different based on factors like age, type of diabetes, and overall health. Your doctor will help you figure out what's right for you. The key is consistency: the closer you can stay to your target range, the better you'll feel.

WHAT IS A1C, ANYWAY?

A1C is a blood test that gives you an average of your blood sugar over the last two to three months. It's kind of like getting your semester grades instead of a pop quiz. If your A1C is high, it means your blood sugar has been running high most of the time. The general goal for people with diabetes is to keep their A1C below 7%. But remember, this is just one piece of the puzzle—don't stress too much over a single number.

WHAT AFFECTS BLOOD SUGAR?

Blood sugar is affected by just about everything: what you eat, how much you move, whether you're stressed out, and even if you have a cold. Here's a quick rundown:

Food

Carbohydrates are the main culprit behind blood sugar spikes. That doesn't mean you have to cut carbs completely, but you'll want to be mindful of what, when, and how much you're eating. (Spoiler: we'll talk more about this in Chapter 5.)

Exercise

Moving your body can help lower blood sugar. When you exercise, your muscles use glucose for energy, which helps bring your levels down. Just be aware that intense exercise can sometimes drop your blood sugar too low—this is where monitoring comes in handy.

Stress

Yep, stress can make your blood sugar go up. When you're stressed, your body releases hormones like cortisol, which can increase your blood sugar. So, the next time you're stuck in traffic or dealing with an annoying email, take a deep breath. Your blood sugar will thank you.

Illness

When you're sick, your body is in a state of stress, which can make your blood sugar rise. Make sure you check your levels more frequently if you're under the weather, and stay hydrated.

Medications

Diabetes meds, obviously, affect blood sugar, but so can other meds, like steroids. Always double-check with your doctor or pharmacist to see how new meds might impact your levels.

HOW OFTEN SHOULD YOU CHECK?

How often you should check your blood sugar depends on a few things: your type of diabetes, your treatment plan, and what your doctor recommends. Here are some general guidelines:

- **Before meals:** This helps you see how well your body handles the food you're about to eat.

- **After meals:** Check about 1-2 hours after eating to see how your body responded.

- **Before bed:** Make sure your levels are stable for a good night's sleep.

- **Whenever you feel "off":** Symptoms like shakiness, sweating, or confusion could mean your blood sugar is out of range, so it's a good idea to check.

Your doctor will give you a more tailored plan based on your needs, but these are good general practices to start with.

HANDLING HIGHS AND LOWS

No matter how diligent you are, you'll likely experience high and low blood sugar at some point. Here's what to do:

High Blood Sugar (Hyperglycemia)

- **Drink water:** Staying hydrated helps your body flush out excess sugar.

- **Exercise:** Light activity can help lower blood sugar—just be cautious if your levels are extremely high (over 300 mg/dL).

- **Follow your treatment plan:** If you're on insulin, follow your doctor's advice on how to bring down high levels.

Low Blood Sugar (Hypoglycemia)

Low blood sugar can make you feel dizzy, sweaty, or even confused. Here's how to handle it:

- **Eat something sugary:** Follow the "15-15 Rule"—have 15 grams of fast-acting carbs (like juice or glucose tablets), wait 15 minutes, and check your blood sugar again.

- **Plan ahead:** Always carry a snack or glucose tablets, just in case.

TAKEAWAY: YOU'RE IN CONTROL

Monitoring your blood sugar may feel like a lot at first, but it'll soon become second nature. And remember, knowledge is power. The more you know about how your body responds to different foods, activities, and situations, the better equipped you'll be to manage your diabetes and keep things in balance.

Next up, we're going to dive into one of the most crucial aspects of diabetes management—what you eat. Get ready for **Chapter 5: Eating Well with Diabetes**, where we'll cover meal planning, carb counting, and all things food.

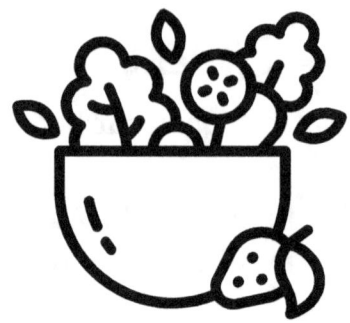

CHAPTER 5:
EATING WELL WITH DIABETES

FOOD: THE FRIEND, NOT THE ENEMY

When you're diagnosed with diabetes, it's easy to start seeing food as the enemy. All those delicious carbs and sweets that you used to eat without a second thought suddenly seem off-limits. But don't worry—you can still enjoy food. In fact, you can eat well and even indulge now and then. The key is learning how to manage what, when, and how much you eat.

Good news: living with diabetes doesn't mean you're saying goodbye to the food you love. It's all about making savvy choices and striking a balance that works for you and your taste buds. Think of this chapter as your guide to building a happy relationship with food again.

UNDERSTANDING CARBS: THE REAL STORY

Carbohydrates (carbs) get a bad rap when it comes to diabetes, but they're not all bad. In fact, carbs are an important part of your diet because they give you energy. The trick is understanding which carbs are friendlier to your blood sugar.

Simple vs. Complex Carbs

There are two main types of carbs: simple and complex.

- **Simple Carbs:** These are quick-digesting carbs, like sugar and white bread. They can spike your blood sugar faster than you can say "chocolate cake." You'll want to limit these.

- **Complex Carbs:** These carbs take longer to break down, which means they give you a slower, more stable rise in blood sugar. Think whole grains, beans, and vegetables.

Choosing complex carbs over simple carbs can help keep your blood sugar in check while still letting you enjoy delicious food.

Fiber: The Carb You Actually Want

Fiber is a type of carb that your body doesn't digest. It helps keep your blood sugar steady, keeps you full, and is generally awesome for your health. Foods like vegetables, fruits, beans, and whole grains are high in fiber. So, go ahead and fill up on these.

CARB COUNTING 101

Carb counting is a handy tool for managing diabetes. It's exactly what it sounds like: you count the grams of carbs you're eating to help keep your blood sugar within your target range. Here's a quick guide:

1. **Know Your Target:** Your doctor or dietitian will give you a target for how many carbs you should eat at each meal and snack.

2. **Read Labels:** Look at the Nutrition Facts on food labels. Pay attention to the "Total Carbohydrates" section—that's the number you want to track.

3. **Subtract the Fiber:** Since fiber doesn't raise blood sugar, you can subtract it from the total carbs. This gives you the "net carbs," which are the carbs that actually affect your blood sugar.

Once you get the hang of it, carb counting becomes second nature. It's all about knowing your limits and enjoying what you eat within those boundaries.

BUILDING A BALANCED PLATE

The easiest way to think about meals with diabetes is to build a balanced plate. This means including a little of everything your body needs: protein, carbs, and healthy fats. Here's a simple formula:

1. **Fill Half Your Plate with Non-Starchy Vegetables:** Veggies like spinach, broccoli, and peppers are low in carbs but packed with nutrients. Plus, they're great for keeping you full.

2. **Fill a Quarter of Your Plate with Lean Protein:** Think chicken, fish, tofu, or beans. Protein helps you feel satisfied and doesn't spike your blood sugar.

3. **Fill a Quarter of Your Plate with Whole Grains or Starchy Veggies:** This could be brown rice, quinoa, sweet potatoes, or whole-grain pasta. These complex carbs give you energy without a huge spike.

4. **Add a Little Healthy Fat:** Top your salad with avocado, drizzle olive oil on your veggies, or toss some nuts into your meal. Fats help you stay full longer and add flavor.

This method keeps things simple while ensuring you're getting a good balance of nutrients.

SNACK SMART

When you have diabetes, snacking is about more than just satisfying cravings. It's also a way to keep your blood sugar stable between meals. The key is to choose snacks that have protein, fiber, or healthy fats—things that don't cause big blood sugar spikes. Here are some snack ideas:

- **Greek yogurt with berries**

- **Apple slices with almond butter**

- **A handful of nuts**

- **Carrot sticks with hummus**

- **Cheese and whole-grain crackers**

Having snack on hand can help prevent those "I'm starving!" moments that lead to overeating. And with snacks like these, you'll be fueling your body with good stuff.

THE POWER OF PORTION CONTROL

Eating well with diabetes doesn't mean you have to give up your favorite foods—it just means you might need to enjoy them in smaller portions. Here are some quick tips for portion control:

- **Use Smaller Plates:** It sounds simple, but it works. A smaller plate makes portions look bigger, which tricks your brain into feeling satisfied with less.

- **Serve Food in the Kitchen:** Instead of putting serving dishes on the table, leave them in the kitchen. It's a subtle reminder to think twice before going back for seconds.

- **Follow the One-Plate Rule:** Limit yourself to one plate of food at each meal. Fill it up with the good stuff, and skip the seconds.

- **Measure Your Carbs:** If you're having rice, pasta, or another carb-heavy food, measure it out before putting it on your plate. A little goes a long way.

With a few simple tricks, portion control can become a habit. It's all about eating mindfully and listening to your body.

NAVIGATING SPECIAL OCCASIONS

Let's be real: you're going to run into birthdays, holidays, and pizza nights. The good news? You don't have to sit these out! Here are some strategies for enjoying special occasions without derailing your blood sugar:

1. **Plan Ahead:** If you know you're going to a party, eat a small, balanced meal beforehand. You'll be less tempted to dive into the chips and dip.

2. **Choose Your Treat:** Go ahead and enjoy a slice of cake or a few bites of your favorite dessert—just skip the sugary drinks or other carb-heavy sides.

3. **Stay Hydrated:** Sometimes, we mistake thirst for hunger. Drink water throughout the event to help keep your blood sugar steady.

4. **Keep Moving:** If you can, take a walk after a big meal. Even a short stroll can help your body process the extra carbs.

With a little planning, you can enjoy life's celebrations while still taking care of your health.

EATING OUT: THE DO'S AND DON'TS

Eating out can be tricky, but it's totally doable. Here are some tips for staying on track when you're at a restaurant:

- **Check the Menu Ahead of Time:** Look up the menu online and choose a healthy option before you arrive. That way, you're not swayed by the sight of cheese fries.

- **Ask for Modifications:** Don't be shy about asking for swaps. Most restaurants are happy to substitute salad for fries or serve your sauce on the side.

- **Watch the Portions:** Restaurant portions are often huge. Consider splitting a meal with a friend or taking half of it home.

- **Skip the Bread Basket:** It's okay to ask the server not to bring it. Out of sight, out of mind!

- **Be Wary of Hidden Sugars:** Dressings, sauces, and marinades can be sugar bombs. Ask for these on the side, or choose simpler options.

Eating out is a part of life, and you can still enjoy it. The key is to make mindful choices and listen to your body.

TAKEAWAY: ENJOY YOUR FOOD, ENJOY YOUR LIFE

Eating well with diabetes is all about balance. You don't have to give up the foods you love, but learning how to eat mindfully and control your portions will help you feel your best. Remember, this is a journey, not a race. You'll have good days and bad days, and that's okay. What matters is that you're making choices that support your health and make you feel good.

Up next, we'll talk about how exercise fits into the picture. It's time for **Chapter 6: Exercise for a Healthy Lifestyle**—get ready to move!

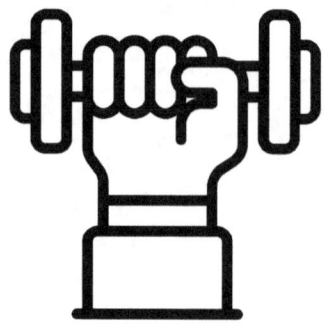

CHAPTER 6:
EXERCISE FOR A HEALTHY LIFESTYLE

WHY EXERCISE MATTERS

By now, you know that managing diabetes isn't just about food and medication—it's also about staying active. Exercise is like a secret weapon for keeping your blood sugar stable, boosting your energy, and even improving your mood. Plus, it has a whole host of other benefits, like reducing stress and helping you sleep better. And the best part? You don't have to turn into a gym rat to see the benefits.

Moving your body, even a little bit each day, can make a big difference. So let's talk about why exercise is so important for diabetes management and how you can find activities you actually enjoy.

HOW EXERCISE AFFECTS BLOOD SUGAR

When you exercise, your muscles use glucose for energy, which helps lower your blood sugar. It's kind of like your muscles are burning off extra fuel. Plus, physical activity makes your cells more sensitive to insulin, which means your body can use insulin more effectively.

But here's a little heads-up: exercise can affect your blood sugar in different ways depending on what type of workout you're doing, how long you're doing it, and what you've eaten before. For instance, a quick walk might lower your blood sugar right away, while a weightlifting session might cause a delayed drop later on. The more you understand how your body responds, the easier it becomes to fit exercise into your routine.

TYPES OF EXERCISE: FINDING YOUR FIT

There are a few main types of exercise, and each one has its own set of benefits. Let's break them down:

1. Aerobic Exercise: The Heart-Pumper

Aerobic exercise, or cardio, is anything that gets your heart rate up. This includes activities like walking, jogging, cycling, swimming, and dancing. Cardio is great for burning calories, improving heart health, and lowering blood sugar.

Goal: Aim for at least 150 minutes of moderate-intensity cardio per week. This could be 30 minutes a day, five days a week.

2. Strength Training: The Muscle-Builder

Strength training involves using resistance (like weights or resistance bands) to build muscle. This is super important for diabetes because more muscle means your body can use glucose more effectively. Strength training can also boost your metabolism, helping you burn more calories even at rest.

Goal: Try to do strength training exercises two to three times a week. You don't need fancy equipment—bodyweight exercises like squats and push-ups work too!

3. Flexibility and Balance: The Unsung Heroes

Activities like yoga, Pilates, and stretching improve flexibility and balance. While they don't burn as many calories, they help with mobility and reduce the risk of injuries. Plus, they're great for relaxation and stress relief, which is always a plus for managing diabetes.

Goal: Incorporate flexibility and balance exercises into your routine a few times a week. Even just a few minutes of stretching each day can make a difference.

STARTING SMALL: BABY STEPS COUNT!

If you're new to exercise, don't feel like you have to dive into a full-blown workout plan right away. Start small. Take a 10-minute walk around the block, try some light stretching in the morning, or dance around your living room to your favorite song. The goal is to find movement that feels good and build from there.

Remember, every bit counts. Even small bursts of activity can help improve your blood sugar and overall health. The key is consistency—try to move a little every day, and before you know it, you'll start feeling the benefits.

MAKING EXERCISE A HABIT

We all know that exercising is easier said than done. Life gets busy, motivation fades, and before you know it, you've skipped a week (or more). The trick to sticking with exercise is to make it a habit. Here are some tips:

- **Find Something You Enjoy:** If you hate running, don't run. Try swimming, biking, or dancing instead. The best exercise is the one you'll actually do.

- **Set Realistic Goals:** Start with small, achievable goals, like walking for 10 minutes a day, and build from there. Celebrate your progress, no matter how small.

- **Schedule It In:** Treat exercise like any other appointment. Put it on your calendar, set reminders, and make it a non-negotiable part of your day.

- **Buddy Up:** Working out with a friend can make exercise more fun and keep you accountable. Plus, it's always nice to have someone to cheer you on.

- **Mix It Up:** Avoid boredom by trying new activities. Take a hike, join a yoga class, or try a new workout video. Variety keeps things interesting.

STAYING SAFE WHILE EXERCISING

Safety first! Before you jump into a new exercise routine, check with your doctor, especially if you're on medication or have any health concerns. Here are some general tips for staying safe:

- **Check Your Blood Sugar:** If you're on insulin or certain diabetes meds, check your blood sugar before and after exercise. This will help you learn how your body responds and prevent lows.

- **Stay Hydrated:** Drink water before, during, and after exercise. Dehydration can mess with your blood sugar levels, so keep a water bottle handy.

- **Listen to Your Body:** Pay attention to how you feel. If you're dizzy, lightheaded, or unusually tired, take a break. It's better to ease into things than to push too hard and risk injury.

- **Wear the Right Shoes:** If you're doing any weight-bearing exercise (like walking or running), make sure you have supportive shoes that fit well. This is especially important for people with diabetes, as foot health is a big deal.

HANDLING EXERCISE HIGHS AND LOWS

Exercise can cause both highs and lows in your blood sugar, so it's good to be prepared. Here's what to watch for:

Exercise-Induced Lows

If your blood sugar drops too low during exercise, you might feel shaky, sweaty, or dizzy. This can happen if you've taken insulin or haven't eaten enough before working out.

- **Quick Fix:** If you feel low, stop exercising and eat or drink something with fast-acting carbs, like juice or glucose tablets. Check your blood sugar again after 15 minutes to make sure it's back in range.

Exercise-Induced Highs

Sometimes, intense exercise can actually raise your blood sugar temporarily, especially if you're doing high-intensity activities like sprinting or heavy lifting. This is usually due to stress hormones kicking in.

- **Quick Fix:** If your blood sugar goes high, take a breather and drink some water. It should come back down on its own. If you're consistently seeing highs, talk to your doctor for advice.

TAKEAWAY:
MAKE MOVEMENT A PART OF YOUR LIFE

Exercise doesn't have to be a chore. Find activities you enjoy, start small, and make movement a regular part of your routine. Remember, the goal is to move your body in a way that feels good, helps manage your blood sugar, and keeps you feeling strong and healthy. And don't forget—it's okay to have fun with it!

Up next, we'll talk about medications and insulin management in **Chapter 7: Medication and Insulin Management**. Understanding how these tools work will give you even more control over your diabetes.

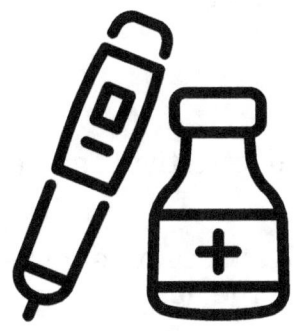

CHAPTER 7:
MEDICATION AND INSULIN MANAGEMENT

MEDICATIONS AND INSULIN: YOUR SECRET WEAPONS

Alright, we've talked about food, exercise, and monitoring your blood sugar. Now it's time to tackle another big piece of the puzzle: medications and insulin. These tools can help you keep your blood sugar in check, prevent complications, and generally make managing diabetes a whole lot easier.

Whether you're taking pills, using insulin, or a combo of both, it's all about finding the right plan for you. This chapter will break down the different types of diabetes medications, how insulin works, and tips for managing everything like a pro.

DIABETES MEDICATIONS 101

Let's start with the basics. There are a few types of diabetes medications out there, and they each work in their own way. Your doctor will prescribe the one that fits best with your type of diabetes, your lifestyle, and your body's needs.

1. Metformin: The First-Line Defender

If you've got Type 2 diabetes, there's a good chance your doctor started you on metformin. It's one of the most commonly prescribed diabetes meds and helps lower blood sugar by reducing the amount of glucose your liver makes and helping your body use insulin more effectively. It's like giving your liver a little nudge to chill out.

- **Pros:** Usually well-tolerated, effective, and often the first choice for Type 2.

- **Cons:** It can cause stomach upset for some people. If this happens, talk to your doctor about adjusting the dose.

2. Sulfonylureas: The Insulin Boosters

These meds (like glipizide and glyburide) help your pancreas pump out more insulin. They can be very effective, especially if your body still makes some insulin on its own.

- **Pros:** Works quickly and can be taken once or twice a day.

- **Cons:** Can sometimes cause low blood sugar, so you'll need to monitor closely.

3. DPP-4 Inhibitors: The Sugar Controllers

DPP-4 inhibitors (like sitagliptin and linagliptin) work by helping your body release more insulin and lowering the amount of glucose your liver releases. They don't cause weight gain and are generally well-tolerated.

- **Pros:** Low risk of hypoglycemia, doesn't usually cause weight gain.

- **Cons:** Can be expensive without insurance coverage.

4. GLP-1 Receptor Agonists: The Appetite Suppressors

These injectable medications (like liraglutide and exenatide) help lower blood sugar by increasing insulin production, reducing glucose release, and slowing down digestion, which can help with weight loss.

- **Pros:** Helps with weight loss, can reduce risk of heart disease.

- **Cons:** Injectables, so they might not be everyone's favorite; can cause nausea.

5. SGLT2 Inhibitors: The Sugar Flushers

These meds (like empagliflozin and canagliflozin) help your kidneys flush out excess sugar through urine. They're known for reducing blood sugar and offering heart and kidney benefits.

- **Pros:** Can lower blood pressure and help with weight loss.

- **Cons:** Can increase risk of urinary tract infections, so hydration is key.

Your doctor will work with you to find the medication or combination that works best for you. Remember, it might take some trial and error to find the right fit, so be patient and keep an open line of communication with your healthcare team.

THE SCOOP ON INSULIN

If you're on insulin, welcome to the club. While taking insulin might sound intimidating, it's a fantastic tool for managing blood sugar. Let's break down the basics.

Types of Insulin

There are several types of insulin, each with a different speed and duration of action:

- **Rapid-Acting Insulin:** Kicks in within 15 minutes and lasts for about 2-4 hours. Great for mealtime control.

- **Short-Acting Insulin:** Takes effect within 30 minutes and lasts about 3-6 hours. Another option for meals.

- **Intermediate-Acting Insulin:** Starts working in 2-4 hours and lasts up to 18 hours. Often used for background control.

- **Long-Acting Insulin:** Takes a few hours to kick in but lasts up to 24 hours. Provides steady, all-day control.

- **Ultra-Long-Acting Insulin:** Lasts longer than 24 hours, providing a consistent level of insulin.

Your doctor will prescribe the type (or types) that fit your lifestyle and blood sugar needs. Sometimes, you might take a long-acting insulin once a day for baseline control and add rapid-acting insulin before meals.

How to Take Insulin

Insulin is typically injected with a syringe, insulin pen, or pump. Here's a quick look at each option:

- **Syringes:** These are the classic choice. You draw up the insulin, inject it, and you're done.

- **Insulin Pens:** Pens are convenient, pre-filled, and easy to carry around. Just dial your dose, inject, and go.

- **Insulin Pumps:** Pumps deliver a steady dose of insulin throughout the day. They're great for people who want a hands-off approach, but they do require some setup and monitoring.

Your healthcare team will show you how to inject insulin, rotate your injection sites, and handle any questions you have. It might seem daunting at first, but you'll get the hang of it quickly.

MANAGING INSULIN AND MEDS LIKE A PRO

Here are some tips for keeping everything on track:

- **Set Reminders:** Use your phone or a pill organizer to remind you when it's time to take your meds or insulin.

- **Monitor Your Blood Sugar:** Keep an eye on your levels, especially if you're adjusting your insulin or starting a new medication.

- **Know the Side Effects:** Make sure you understand the potential side effects of any medication you're taking. That way, you'll know what's normal and when to call your doctor.

- **Carry a Snack:** If you're on insulin or sulfonylureas, always have a quick source of carbs (like juice or glucose tablets) in case your blood sugar drops.

WHAT IF YOU MISS A DOSE?

It happens. You're only human! If you miss a dose of medication, don't double up. Instead, check with your doctor or pharmacist about what to do next. For insulin, it depends on when you missed the dose and your current blood sugar levels. When in doubt, reach out to your healthcare team.

TAKEAWAY: MEDS AND INSULIN ARE PART OF YOUR TOOLKIT

Think of medications and insulin as your trusty sidekicks on this diabetes journey. They're not signs of weakness—quite the opposite! They're the tools that help you keep your blood sugar in check, dodge complications, and keep living your best life. And remember, your healthcare team is there to help you navigate this process. Don't be afraid to ask questions, and keep experimenting until you find what works best for you.

Up next, we'll explore how to manage potential complications and stay healthy in **Chapter 8: Managing Complications and Staying Healthy**.

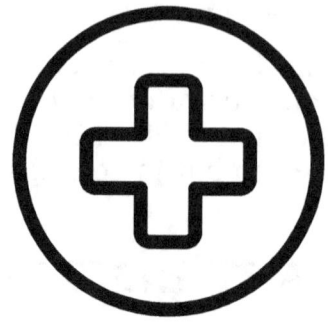

CHAPTER 8:
MANAGING COMPLICATIONS AND STAYING HEALTHY

PREVENTION IS KEY

Managing diabetes isn't just about keeping your blood sugar in check today—it's also about taking steps to stay healthy down the road. With diabetes, there's a higher risk for complications like heart disease, kidney issues, nerve damage, and vision problems. But here's the good news: with proper care, you can avoid or minimize these complications. This chapter will show you how to stay ahead of the game and keep your body running smoothly.

KEEPING YOUR HEART HEALTHY

Heart disease is one of the most common complications associated with diabetes, but don't let that scare you. By making heart health a priority, you can greatly reduce your risk. Here's what you need to know:

Watch Your Blood Pressure

High blood pressure and diabetes often go hand-in-hand, and together they can increase your risk for heart disease. Keeping your blood pressure within a healthy range (usually below 140/90 mmHg) is key. Your doctor will monitor this at your checkups, but it's also something you can track at home with a blood pressure monitor.

Control Your Cholesterol

When your cholesterol is out of whack, it can lead to clogged arteries and heart problems. Keeping both your LDL (bad cholesterol) and HDL (good cholesterol) in check helps protect your heart. Your doctor may prescribe medication, or you may be able to manage it through diet and exercise.

Stay Active and Eat Right

We've talked about exercise and diet already, but here's where they really come into play. Moving your body regularly and eating a balanced diet full of fruits, veggies, and whole grains can do wonders for your heart.

PROTECTING YOUR KIDNEYS

Your kidneys work hard to filter waste from your blood, and diabetes can put extra strain on them. Over time, high blood sugar can damage the tiny blood vessels in your kidneys, leading to a condition called diabetic nephropathy. But you can help keep your kidneys healthy with a few simple steps:

- **Monitor Your Blood Sugar:** Keeping your blood sugar within your target range reduces the strain on your kidneys.

- **Stay Hydrated:** Drinking plenty of water helps your kidneys do their job. Aim for at least eight glasses a day.

- **Get Regular Kidney Function Tests:** Your doctor will likely order tests to check how well your kidneys are working. These include a urine test to check for protein and a blood test to measure your kidney function (called a GFR test).

If your doctor does detect early signs of kidney issues, don't panic—there are medications and lifestyle changes that can help protect your kidneys and prevent further damage.

CARING FOR YOUR EYES

Diabetes can affect your vision, so it's important to keep an eye (pun intended) on your eye health. High blood sugar can damage the blood vessels in your retina, leading to a condition called diabetic retinopathy. Regular eye exams are your best defense against vision problems.

Annual Eye Exams

Even if your vision seems fine, make it a point to see an eye doctor (an ophthalmologist or optometrist) once a year. They'll check for signs of diabetic retinopathy and other eye issues, like cataracts and glaucoma, which are more common in people with diabetes.

Control Your Blood Sugar and Blood Pressure

Keeping your blood sugar and blood pressure under control reduces the risk of eye complications. The healthier your blood vessels, the better for your eyes.

TAKING CARE OF YOUR FEET

Foot care might not be the first thing you think about when it comes to diabetes, but it's actually really important. High blood sugar can lead to nerve damage, called neuropathy, which makes it hard to feel cuts or sores on your feet. Left untreated, minor issues can become big problems.

Inspect Your Feet Daily

Make it a habit to check your feet every day for cuts, blisters, redness, or swelling. Use a mirror if needed, or ask a family member to help.

Keep Your Feet Clean and Dry

Wash your feet daily with warm water (not hot!), and dry them thoroughly, especially between the toes. Moisture can lead to infections, so make sure your feet stay dry.

Choose the Right Footwear

Wear comfortable, well-fitting shoes that protect your feet. Avoid going barefoot, even indoors, as it's easy to step on something sharp without realizing it.

If you notice any changes or have concerns about your feet, don't hesitate to reach out to your doctor or podiatrist. It's better to catch issues early than to wait until they become serious.

NERVE HEALTH AND NEUROPATHY

Diabetes can affect the nerves in your body, leading to neuropathy. The most common form is peripheral neuropathy, which affects the hands and feet. Symptoms include tingling, numbness, and pain. While neuropathy can't always be reversed, managing your blood sugar and taking care of your health can prevent it from getting worse.

Pay Attention to Symptoms

If you notice any unusual sensations in your hands or feet—like tingling, burning, or numbness—let your doctor know. They can recommend treatments to help manage symptoms.

Manage Your Blood Sugar

Keeping your blood sugar within your target range is the best way to protect your nerves. The more stable your levels, the lower the risk of nerve damage.

Consider Supplements

Some people find relief from neuropathy symptoms with supplements like alpha-lipoic acid, vitamin B12, or fish oil. Talk to your doctor before starting any new supplement to make sure it's safe for you.

TAKEAWAY: YOU'RE IN CONTROL OF YOUR HEALTH

Sure, thinking about diabetes complications might feel like facing the boogeyman, but here's the thing—you've got more power to protect your health than you might think. By staying on top of your blood sugar, getting regular checkups, and paying attention to your body, you can prevent or catch complications early. The key is to be proactive—your health is worth the effort.

In the next chapter, we'll dive into **Emotional and Mental Well-being**. Taking care of your mind is just as important as taking care of your body, and we'll explore ways to keep your spirits high as you navigate life with diabetes.

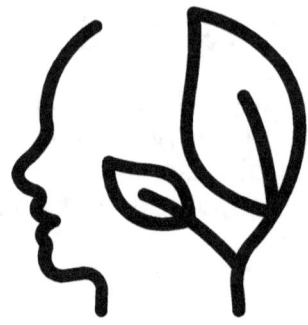

CHAPTER 9:
EMOTIONAL AND MENTAL WELL-BEING

WHY YOUR MENTAL HEALTH MATTERS

Living with diabetes can be challenging—not just physically but also mentally. When you're constantly keeping track of blood sugar, watching what you eat, and worrying about complications, it's easy to feel stressed, overwhelmed, or even anxious. Let's face it: managing diabetes is like having a side gig you didn't sign up for. And yes, it can definitely weigh on your mental health.

But here's the good news: prioritizing your emotional well-being is one of the best things you can do for yourself. Not only will it help you feel better, but a positive outlook and effective stress management can also make managing diabetes easier. In this chapter, we'll explore ways to stay mentally strong, cope with the ups and downs, and take care of your mind as well as your body.

DEALING WITH DIABETES BURNOUT

"Diabetes burnout" is a real thing, and it happens when the daily grind of managing diabetes starts to feel like too much. You might feel tired of checking your blood sugar, fed up with meal planning, or frustrated with all the doctor's appointments. And you know what? That's totally normal.

Everyone gets burned out sometimes. The important thing is to recognize it and take steps to manage it. Here are some strategies:

- **Take a Break:** You don't have to do everything perfectly all the time. Give yourself permission to take a step back. If you miss a blood sugar check or have a day where you eat more carbs than usual, it's okay. Just get back on track the next day.

- **Focus on Small Wins:** When things feel overwhelming, set small, achievable goals. Celebrate little victories like choosing a healthy snack, going for a walk, or taking your meds on time. These small wins add up and remind you that you're making progress.

- **Connect with Others:** Talking to other people with diabetes can be a great way to cope with burnout. They understand what you're going through and can offer support, advice, or just a listening ear.

COPING WITH STRESS AND ANXIETY

Stress is a part of life, but it can be especially challenging when you have diabetes. Stress hormones like cortisol can raise your blood sugar, which is the last thing you need. So, finding ways to manage stress is key to keeping both your mind and body in good shape.

Here are some strategies to help you cope:

1. Practice Relaxation Techniques

Simple techniques like deep breathing, progressive muscle relaxation, and guided imagery can help calm your mind and reduce stress. Even a few minutes of deep breathing can make a difference.

2. Get Moving

Exercise is one of the best stress-busters out there. Physical activity releases endorphins (the feel-good hormones) and helps your body burn off stress. Whether it's a walk around the block, a dance party in your living room, or a yoga class, find something you enjoy and make it a regular part of your routine.

3. Talk to Someone

Sometimes, talking things out can make a world of difference. Whether it's a friend, family member, or therapist, don't be afraid to reach out. A mental health professional can help you develop coping strategies and provide support when you need it.

4. Make Time for Fun

Life with diabetes can feel serious, but it's important to make time for things that make you happy. Whether it's a hobby, a creative outlet, or spending time with loved ones, do what you love and make it a priority.

RECOGNIZING AND MANAGING DIABETES-RELATED DEPRESSION

It's not uncommon for people with diabetes to experience depression. Dealing with a chronic condition can be exhausting, and the added burden of managing diabetes can sometimes lead to feelings of sadness or hopelessness. If you're experiencing symptoms of depression, you're not alone—and there's help available.

Here are some signs of depression to watch for:

- Persistent sadness or feeling down most of the day

- Loss of interest in activities you used to enjoy

- Changes in appetite or sleep patterns

- Feelings of worthlessness or guilt

- Difficulty concentrating or making decisions

- Thoughts of self-harm or suicide

If you're experiencing any of these symptoms, reach out to a mental health professional. There's no shame in asking for help, and there are effective treatments available, like therapy and medication. Taking care of your mental health is just as important as taking care of your physical health.

BUILDING RESILIENCE

Resilience is the ability to bounce back from challenges, and it's a skill you can develop over time. Living with diabetes can be tough, but building resilience can help you handle whatever comes your way.

Here are some ways to boost your resilience:

- **Stay Positive:** This doesn't mean pretending everything is fine when it's not, but it does mean focusing on the good things in your life. Practice gratitude by writing down a few things you're thankful for each day.

- **Set Realistic Goals:** Break your goals down into manageable steps, and don't be too hard on yourself if things don't go perfectly. Progress, not perfection, is what matters.

- **Build a Support System:** Surround yourself with people who lift you up. Whether it's family, friends, or a diabetes support group, having a network of support makes all the difference.

- **Practice Self-Compassion:** Be kind to yourself. It's easy to beat yourself up over setbacks, but remember that you're doing your best. Treat yourself with the same compassion you'd offer a friend.

MINDFULNESS AND MEDITATION

Mindfulness is all about being present in the moment, and it can be a powerful tool for managing stress and improving your mental well-being. Meditation, a form of mindfulness, can help you quiet your mind and focus on the here and now.

If you're new to mindfulness or meditation, start small. Spend a few minutes each day focusing on your breathing, or try a guided meditation app. With practice, you might find that these techniques help you feel more centered and better equipped to handle whatever diabetes throws your way.

TAKEAWAY: YOUR MIND MATTERS

Your mental health is just as important as your physical health, especially when it comes to managing diabetes. By recognizing signs of stress, burnout, or depression and taking proactive steps to care for your emotional well-being, you're setting yourself up for success. Remember, it's okay to ask for help, and taking time for self-care is essential.

Next, we'll explore how to live a full, happy life with diabetes in **Chapter 10: Living a Full Life with Diabetes**. It's all about enjoying life to the fullest, diabetes and all.

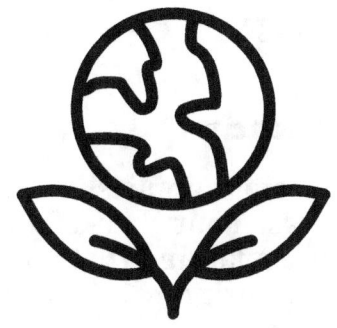

CHAPTER 10:
LIVING A FULL LIFE WITH DIABETES

EMBRACE THE POSSIBILITIES

Yes, diabetes is along for the ride, but it doesn't get to steer. Armed with the right mindset, a little know-how, and plenty of support, you can absolutely live a life that's full of joy, action, and adventure. Whether it's traveling, pursuing your passions, or spending time with loved ones, diabetes doesn't have to hold you back.

This chapter is all about getting out there and enjoying life, with a few practical tips on how to navigate everyday situations with confidence. Let's dive in and explore how to make the most of life, diabetes and all.

TRAVELING WITH DIABETES

Whether you're planning a weekend getaway or a trip around the world, diabetes shouldn't stop you from seeing the sights. With a little extra planning, you can travel just about anywhere. Here are some tips to make traveling with diabetes a breeze:

1. Plan Ahead

Pack a travel kit with all your diabetes essentials: medications, insulin, glucose meter, test strips, and a stash of low-blood-sugar snacks. Bring more supplies than you think you'll need—you never know when a flight might get delayed or plans might change.

2. Keep Your Supplies Handy

When flying, keep all your diabetes supplies in your carry-on bag. That way, you'll have them with you in case your checked luggage goes missing. Also, pack a letter from your doctor explaining that you have diabetes, just in case you need to show it at airport security.

3. Adjust for Time Zones

If you're crossing time zones, talk to your doctor about how to adjust your medication schedule. Insulin timing might need a tweak, so having a plan in place can help you avoid surprises.

4. Stay Hydrated and Move Around

Long flights or road trips can increase the risk of blood clots, so make it a point to drink plenty of water and move around regularly. Flex your legs, stretch, or take a quick walk up and down the aisle.

5. Have a Backup Plan

Things don't always go as planned, especially when you're traveling. Bring extra prescriptions, and know where to find the nearest pharmacy at your destination. With a little preparation, you'll be ready for anything.

NAVIGATING SOCIAL SITUATIONS

Life is full of social events—family gatherings, parties, work events, and more. And yes, you can enjoy these moments while managing your diabetes. Here are some strategies for handling social situations without stressing about your blood sugar:

1. Don't Be Shy About Your Needs

It's okay to let people know you have diabetes. You don't have to make a big announcement, but if someone offers you a sugary drink or extra dessert, feel free to politely decline or explain that you're watching your blood sugar.

2. Make Smart Choices at Buffets and Potlucks

When faced with a spread of food, start by loading up on veggies and lean proteins. Then, choose a few carb-rich foods in small portions. And remember, it's perfectly fine to enjoy a treat—just keep portions in check.

3. BYO Snacks

If you're unsure what food will be available, bring your own diabetes-friendly snacks. This way, you'll always have something safe to eat and won't have to worry about feeling deprived.

4. Keep an Eye on Your Blood Sugar

Social events can be unpredictable, so keep your glucose meter handy and check your blood sugar as needed. It's better to be proactive and make adjustments if you notice your levels are off.

ENJOYING SPECIAL OCCASIONS

Birthdays, holidays, and celebrations are part of life, and they're meant to be enjoyed. You can still participate in these moments with a few smart strategies:

- **Plan Ahead:** If you know you're attending an event with lots of treats, eat a balanced meal beforehand. This way, you'll feel less tempted to overindulge.

- **Choose Your Treats Wisely:** Have a small slice of cake, a piece of chocolate, or whatever you love. The key is moderation—enjoy it mindfully and then get back to your regular routine.

- **Stay Active:** If you can, go for a walk after a big meal or celebration. This helps your body process any extra carbs and keeps your blood sugar stable.

Celebrations are about more than just food—they're about spending time with people you care about. Focus on the moments, not just the menu, and you'll create wonderful memories without feeling deprived.

HOBBIES AND PHYSICAL ACTIVITIES

Diabetes doesn't mean you have to give up activities you enjoy. In fact, hobbies and physical activities can be great for managing stress, staying active, and feeling good. Whether you love hiking, dancing, gardening, or playing sports, there's no reason to let diabetes hold you back.

Here are some tips for staying active in ways that work for you:

- **Listen to Your Body:** Be mindful of how you're feeling, and don't push yourself too hard. Check your blood sugar before and after physical activities, and keep a snack handy in case you need it.

- **Set Realistic Goals:** If you're starting a new activity, set small goals and build up gradually. Celebrate your progress, no matter how big or small.

- **Stay Hydrated:** Drink water before, during, and after activities to keep your body fueled and your blood sugar stable.

- **Have Fun:** Choose activities that you genuinely enjoy. The more fun you have, the more likely you'll stick with it.

RELATIONSHIPS AND SUPPORT

Diabetes doesn't just affect you—it can impact your relationships with friends, family, and even coworkers. The key is open communication and finding a support system that works for you.

- **Educate Your Loved Ones:** Help your family and friends understand what diabetes is and how they can support you. Share with them what you're going through, and let them know how they can help.

- **Lean on Others:** It's okay to ask for help. Whether it's asking a friend to join you for a walk or sharing your experiences with a diabetes support group, connecting with others can make a big difference.

- **Set Boundaries:** Sometimes, people mean well but don't fully understand what you're going through. If someone gives unsolicited advice or comments on what you're eating, it's okay to politely set boundaries. You're the expert on your own body.

Building a network of supportive people who understand your journey can help you feel more confident and empowered.

TAKEAWAY: DIABETES DOESN'T DEFINE YOU

You are so much more than your diabetes. It's just one part of your life, and it doesn't have to stop you from doing the things you love. By staying active, planning ahead, and finding the right support, you can live a full, vibrant life with diabetes. Enjoy the journey, embrace the possibilities, and remember that diabetes is just a small part of who you are.

Next, we'll focus on building long-term healthy habits in **Chapter 11: Building Long-term Healthy Habits**. These habits will help you stay on track and feel your best for years to come.

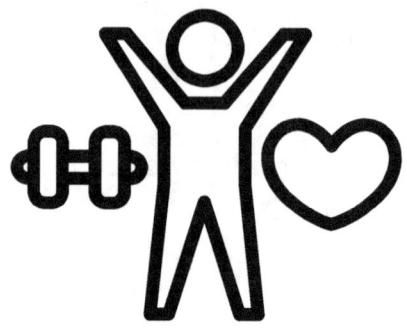

CHAPTER 11:
BUILDING LONG-TERM HEALTHY HABITS

SMALL CHANGES, BIG IMPACT

Living well with diabetes isn't about quick fixes or temporary solutions—it's about building habits that will keep you healthy for the long haul. The good news? You don't have to make big, dramatic changes all at once. In fact, small, consistent steps are the secret to long-term success. This chapter is all about helping you create healthy habits that fit your life, are sustainable, and will keep you feeling your best.

SETTING REALISTIC GOALS

We all start out with big dreams, like totally transforming our lives by next week. But here's the scoop: aiming too high too soon often leads straight to burnout city. Let's keep it real and set goals you can actually stick with. Instead, set realistic, achievable goals that you can build on over time.

1. Start Small

Choose one habit to focus on, like drinking more water, going for a daily walk, or eating more vegetables. Once you've got that down, add another habit. Remember, progress is progress—no matter how small.

2. Be Specific

Vague goals like "exercise more" or "eat better" can be hard to stick to. Instead, be specific: "I will go for a 10-minute walk after dinner," or "I will eat a salad with lunch three days a week." The clearer your goal, the easier it is to follow through.

3. Track Your Progress

Keep a journal, use an app, or mark off days on a calendar—whatever helps you see your progress. Tracking can be incredibly motivating, and it helps you see how far you've come.

BUILDING HABITS THAT STICK

We all know how easy it is to start a new habit, only to give up a few weeks later. Here are some tips for making your new habits stick:

1. Make It Part of Your Routine

The more a habit feels like a natural part of your day, the more likely you are to stick with it. Tie new habits to something you already do. For example, if you want to take your medication consistently, do it right after brushing your teeth in the morning.

2. Set Up Reminders

It's easy to forget new habits, especially when life gets busy. Set reminders on your phone, leave sticky notes where you'll see them, or ask a friend to check in with you. Reminders are like little nudges that keep you on track.

3. Reward Yourself

Positive reinforcement goes a long way. Treat yourself to something you enjoy after a week of sticking to your habit. It could be a favorite snack, a relaxing bath, or a fun activity. Knowing there's a reward at the end can help you stay motivated.

THE POWER OF ROUTINE

Routines create a sense of structure and make healthy choices easier. When you have a routine, you're less likely to make impulsive decisions, like skipping a workout or reaching for an unhealthy snack. Here's how to build a routine that supports your health:

- **Morning Routine:** Start your day with a glass of water, a healthy breakfast, and a quick stretch. Setting a positive tone in the morning can make a big difference in your day.

- **Mealtime Routine:** Plan and prep your meals as much as possible. This helps you make healthier choices and prevents last-minute, less healthy options.

- **Evening Routine:** Wind down with a relaxing activity, check your blood sugar if needed, and prepare for the next day. A consistent bedtime routine also helps improve sleep quality.

Your routine doesn't have to be rigid or complicated. The key is consistency—doing small things every day that help you feel good and stay on track.

STAYING MOTIVATED OVER THE LONG HAUL

Motivation can come and go, especially when it comes to lifestyle changes. Here are some ways to stay motivated, even when the initial excitement wears off:

1. Remember Your "Why"

Why do you want to build these habits? Is it to feel better, have more energy, or reduce your risk of complications? Whatever your reasons, keep them front and center. Write them down, and revisit them often.

2. Surround Yourself with Support

Having a support system can make a huge difference. Share your goals with friends, family, or a diabetes support group. Their encouragement can help you stay focused, especially on tough days.

3. Don't Be Too Hard on Yourself

No one is perfect, and you're bound to have slip-ups. When that happens, be kind to yourself. Reflect on what happened, learn from it, and get back on track. Building habits is a journey, not a sprint.

4. Celebrate Your Wins

Take time to celebrate your progress. Whether it's a big milestone or a small achievement, give yourself credit for the work you've put in. Recognizing your efforts keeps you motivated and reminds you that you're making a difference.

THE ROLE OF ACCOUNTABILITY

Accountability can be a powerful motivator. Knowing that someone else is watching your progress or that you have a check-in coming up can keep you on track. Here are a few ways to stay accountable:

- **Check-Ins with Your Healthcare Team:** Regular appointments with your doctor or diabetes educator can help you stay focused on your health goals. They can offer guidance, track your progress, and adjust your plan as needed.

- **Accountability Partner:** Find a friend, family member, or fellow person with diabetes who can be your accountability partner. Share your goals, check in with each other regularly, and celebrate each other's successes.

- **Online Communities:** There are plenty of online diabetes communities and forums where you can connect with others who are on the same journey. These communities can provide support, encouragement, and tips for staying on track.

BUILDING A HEALTHY MINDSET

A big part of building long-term habits is developing a mindset that supports your goals. This means embracing progress over perfection, being patient with yourself, and believing in your ability to change.

- **Focus on Progress, Not Perfection:** It's easy to get discouraged if you're not perfect. Remember that every small step counts. Focus on how far you've come, not on how far you have to go.

- **Practice Patience:** Real change takes time, and there will be ups and downs along the way. Be patient with yourself, and trust that with consistency, you'll see results.

- **Believe in Yourself:** You are capable of making positive changes, and you deserve to feel good. Believe in your ability to stick with your habits, even when it's challenging.

TAKEAWAY: HABITS FOR A LIFETIME

Building long-term healthy habits is all about taking small steps, staying consistent, and being kind to yourself. Remember, these habits aren't about restriction or deprivation—they're about creating a life that makes you feel your best. Keep moving forward, celebrate your progress, and know that each day is a new opportunity to take care of yourself.

Next up, we'll wrap things up in **Chapter 12: Moving Forward with Confidence**, where we'll review everything you've learned and talk about how to keep thriving with diabetes.

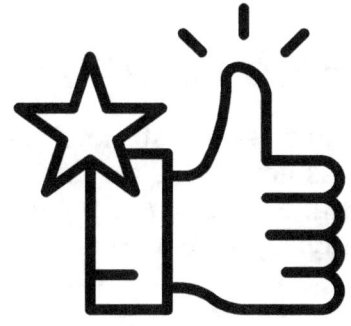

CHAPTER 12:
MOVING FORWARD WITH CONFIDENCE

YOU'VE GOT THIS

Congratulations! You've made it to the end of the book, and now you're equipped with the knowledge and tools to take on life with diabetes. From understanding the basics of diabetes and learning how to manage your blood sugar, to embracing a healthy lifestyle and building long-term habits—you're ready to move forward with confidence.

Diabetes might have crashed the party uninvited, but you're handling it like a pro. You've proven you can roll with whatever life throws your way. You've got the skills, the support, and the resilience to thrive. This chapter is all about keeping that momentum going, staying motivated, and continuing to live a full, wonderful life.

EMBRACE YOUR NEW NORMAL

By now, you've probably realized that living with diabetes isn't a one-time thing—it's an ongoing journey. The good news is that you're not just surviving, you're thriving. You've adapted, you've learned, and you've made changes that will benefit you for years to come.

Embrace your new normal with pride. You've worked hard to get here, and you've earned the right to live life on your terms. Remember, diabetes is just one part of who you are. It doesn't define you, and it doesn't limit your potential. You are so much more than your diagnosis.

KEEP LEARNING AND GROWING

Diabetes management isn't static—it's something you'll continue to learn about and adjust over time. As you move forward, remember that it's okay to keep learning and adapting. New research, treatments, and technologies are always emerging, and staying informed can help you stay on top of your health.

Here are some ways to keep learning:

- **Stay in Touch with Your Healthcare Team:** Regular check-ins with your doctor, dietitian, or diabetes educator can help you stay up-to-date on the latest developments and ensure your care plan is still working for you.

- **Seek Out Resources:** There are countless books, podcasts, and online resources dedicated to diabetes management. Keep exploring and expanding your knowledge.

- **Connect with the Diabetes Community:** Joining a diabetes support group or online community can help you stay motivated and learn from others who are on a similar journey. Plus, it's a great way to make new friends who understand what you're going through.

CELEBRATE YOUR PROGRESS

Take a moment to reflect on everything you've accomplished. Managing diabetes takes hard work, and you've made incredible progress. Celebrate the small wins, the big wins, and everything in between. Recognize your resilience, your determination, and your commitment to your health.

Remember, every step forward is worth celebrating. You've shown that you can handle challenges and make positive changes, and that's something to be proud of.

LOOKING AHEAD

Life with diabetes is full of opportunities. Whether it's trying a new exercise routine, experimenting with healthy recipes, or exploring new places, the future is yours to shape. Don't let diabetes hold you back from pursuing your dreams and passions. Embrace new experiences, stay curious, and keep pushing yourself to grow.

As you look ahead, remember that you're not alone. You've got a support system, a toolkit of skills, and the strength to keep moving forward. With every day, you're building a healthier, happier, and more fulfilling life.

TAKEAWAY:
YOU ARE CAPABLE, RESILIENT, AND STRONG

Living with diabetes isn't easy, but you've proven that you're capable, resilient, and strong. You've taken on the challenges, learned valuable lessons, and built a life that supports your health and well-being. As you move forward, keep believing in yourself and your ability to live a wonderful life with diabetes.

This journey is yours to continue, and I have no doubt that you'll keep thriving. So go out there, live fully, and remember that you've got this. You're ready for whatever comes next.

FINAL THOUGHTS

Thank you for letting me be a part of your journey. It's been a privilege to share these tools and insights with you. Living with diabetes is a unique experience, and no two journeys are the same. But wherever your path takes you, know that you have everything you need to live a vibrant, fulfilling life.

Here's to you, your health, and the many amazing adventures that lie ahead. Stay strong, stay positive, and keep moving forward with confidence. You've got this.

REFERENCES

- *American Diabetes Association. (2021). Standards of Medical Care in Diabetes—2021.*

- *Centers for Disease Control and Prevention. (2020). National Diabetes Statistics Report.*

- *National Institute of Diabetes and Digestive and Kidney Diseases. (2020). Diabetes Overview.*

- *American Heart Association. (2019). Diabetes and Heart Disease.*

- *Mayo Clinic Staff. (2021). Diabetes Diet: Create Your Healthy-Eating Plan.*

ATTRIBUTIONS
FOR USE OF ALL THE BEAUTIFUL ICONS

Chapter 1
By **WEBTECHOPS LLP** from <u>thenounproject.com</u>

Chapter 2
By **Romaldon** from <u>thenounproject.com</u>

Chapter 3
By **Dewi Novita Sari** from <u>thenounproject.com</u>

Chapter 4
By **Andre Buand** from <u>thenounproject.com</u>

Chapter 5
By **Iconbunny** from <u>thenounproject.com</u>

Chapter 6
By **Farit Al Fauzi** from <u>thenounproject.com</u>

Chapter 7
By **Icon From Us** from <u>thenounproject.com</u>

Chapter 8
By **Mada Creative** from <u>thenounproject.com</u>

Chapter 9
By **ridhobadal** from <u>thenounproject.com</u>

Chapter 10
By **Numeralia Vita Zein** from <u>thenounproject.com</u>

Chapter 11
By **Lars Meiertoberens** from <u>thenounproject.com</u>

Chapter 12
By **SAM Designs** from <u>thenounproject.com</u>